INTRODUCTION

The Metabolic Confusion Diet is a type of diet that is designed to promote weight loss by constantly varying the type and amount of food eaten on a daily basis. The diet is based on the theory that by constantly changing the macronutrient ratios and caloric intake, the body is less likely to adapt to a fixed pattern of eating, which can cause a plateau in weight loss.

The diet typically involves four phases of different caloric intake and macronutrient ratios, which are rotated throughout the week. The phases can range from high-carbohydrate and low-fat to low-carbohydrate and high-fat. By constantly changing the body's diet, the metabolic confusion diet aims to prevent the body from adapting to a fixed pattern of eating, thereby increasing metabolism and promoting weight loss.

One of the key principles of the metabolic confusion diet is calorie cycling, which involves varying the number of calories consumed each day. This can be achieved by consuming more calories on some days and fewer calories on others, or by alternating high-calorie and low-calorie days. The idea behind calorie cycling is that it can prevent the body from adapting to a fixed calorie intake, thereby keeping the metabolism elevated and promoting weight loss.

Another important aspect of the metabolic confusion diet

is the emphasis on whole, unprocessed foods. The diet encourages the consumption of lean protein, complex carbohydrates, and healthy fats while avoiding processed foods, sugar, and refined carbohydrates.

Proponents of the metabolic confusion diet claim that it can help individuals achieve sustainable weight loss while also improving overall health markers such as blood sugar, cholesterol, and blood pressure. However, it is important to note that the diet may not be suitable for everyone, particularly those with certain medical conditions or dietary restrictions.

Overall, the metabolic confusion diet is an approach to weight loss that involves cycling between different phases of eating to boost metabolism and promote weight loss. While there is some evidence to support its effectiveness, it is important to consult with a healthcare professional before embarking on any new diet or weight loss plan.

CHAPTER ONE

*Overview of Metabolic
Confusion Diet*

Brief History Of The Diet

The Metabolic Confusion Diet is a relatively new diet that has gained popularity in recent years, but its principles have been used in bodybuilding and fitness circles for many years. The concept of calorie cycling, for example, has been used as a way to boost metabolism and promote muscle growth.

The idea behind calorie cycling is that by varying the number of calories consumed each day, the body is less likely to adapt to a fixed calorie intake, which can cause a plateau in weight loss. The Metabolic Confusion Diet takes this idea further by incorporating different phases of eating, which are rotated throughout the week.

The concept of metabolic confusion is based on the idea that the body is designed to adapt to changes in diet and exercise, which can cause weight loss to plateau. By constantly varying the type and amount of food eaten on a daily basis, the Metabolic Confusion Diet aims to prevent the body from adapting to a fixed pattern of eating, thereby keeping the metabolism elevated and promoting weight loss.

The Metabolic Confusion Diet was first popularized by fitness expert Jay Cardiello in his 2012 book "Cardio Core 4x4: The 20-Minute, No-Gym Workout That Will Transform Your Body!" In the book, Cardiello described how varying the intensity and duration of workouts could confuse the body's metabolism and lead to greater weight loss.

Cardiello later expanded on this concept and developed the Metabolic Confusion Diet, which involves four phases of different caloric intake and macronutrient ratios, which are rotated throughout the week. These phases can range from high-carbohydrate and low-fat to low-carbohydrate and high-fat.

While the Metabolic Confusion Diet is a relatively new concept, it has gained popularity among fitness enthusiasts and has been promoted by several other fitness experts and celebrities. Proponents of the diet claim that it can help individuals achieve sustainable weight loss while also improving overall health markers such as blood sugar, cholesterol, and blood pressure.

However, it is important to note that the Metabolic Confusion Diet may not be suitable for everyone, particularly those with certain medical conditions or dietary restrictions. As with any new diet or weight loss plan, it is important to consult with a healthcare professional before embarking on the Metabolic Confusion Diet.

Explanation Of How The Diet Works

The Metabolic Confusion Diet works by cycling through different phases of calorie intake and macronutrient ratios throughout the week, with the goal of keeping the metabolism elevated and promoting weight loss.

The diet typically involves four phases that are rotated throughout the week. These phases can vary in their caloric intake, as well as in their macronutrient ratios. For example, one phase might involve high carbohydrate and low fat intake, while another phase might involve low carbohydrate and high fat intake.

The idea behind this cycling of calorie and macronutrient intake is to prevent the body from adapting to a fixed pattern of eating. When the body is exposed to the same pattern of eating every day, it can adapt by slowing down the metabolism and reducing energy expenditure. By constantly varying the type and amount of food consumed, the Metabolic Confusion Diet aims to prevent the body from adapting in this way, thereby keeping the metabolism elevated and promoting weight loss.

Additionally, the Metabolic Confusion Diet encourages regular exercise as a way to further boost the metabolism and promote weight loss. The diet recommends a combination of resistance training and cardiovascular exercise, with an emphasis on high-intensity interval training (HIIT) to maximize fat burning and calorie expenditure.

Overall, the Metabolic Confusion Diet works by constantly varying the type and amount of food consumed, as well as by incorporating regular exercise to keep the metabolism elevated and promote weight loss. While its effectiveness is still being studied, many individuals have reported success with the diet in achieving sustainable weight loss and improving overall health markers.

Common mistakes to avoid

There are a few common mistakes that people can make when following the Metabolic Confusion Diet. These include:

1. **Not following the phases correctly:** Each phase of the diet has specific guidelines for what to eat and when. It's important to follow these guidelines carefully to get the most benefit from the diet.

2. **Not drinking enough water:** Adequate hydration is important for overall health and can also help with weight loss. It's recommended to drink at least 8 glasses of water per day.

3. **Not getting enough sleep:** Sleep is essential for overall health and can also impact weight loss. It's recommended to get 7-9 hours of sleep per night.

4. **Overeating during the high calorie phase:** While the high calorie phase can be tempting, it's important not to overeat and to stick to the recommended portion sizes.

5. **Not incorporating exercise:** Exercise is an

important component of the diet and can help with weight loss and overall health. It's recommended to incorporate both cardio and strength training exercises into your routine.

6. **Not tracking progress:** It's important to track progress and make adjustments as needed to ensure success on the diet. This can include tracking weight loss, body measurements, and changes in energy levels and overall health.

Potential Side Effects Of The Diet

While the Metabolic Confusion Diet is generally considered safe for most healthy individuals, there are some potential side effects that should be considered.

One potential side effect is a decrease in energy levels, especially during the initial phases when calories are restricted. This can be alleviated by making sure to eat enough calories and nutrients, and also by incorporating regular exercise into the plan.

Another potential side effect is hunger and cravings, particularly during the low-calorie days. It's important to stay hydrated and choose nutrient-dense foods to help keep feelings of hunger at bay.

In some cases, individuals may experience digestive issues such as bloating, constipation, or diarrhea due to changes in their diet. This can often be managed by gradually introducing new foods and increasing fiber intake.

Finally, it's worth noting that any major dietary changes

can potentially impact mental health and mood. Some individuals may experience irritability, mood swings, or difficulty focusing during the initial phases of the diet. Staying mindful, practicing self-care, and seeking support from a healthcare provider or counselor can be helpful in managing any mental health concerns that may arise.

Who Should Not Follow The Diet

The Metabolic Confusion Diet is generally safe for most healthy individuals, but there are some groups of people who should avoid following this diet. These include:

1. **Pregnant or nursing women:** The diet may not provide enough nutrients for the needs of a developing fetus or a nursing baby.

2. **Children and adolescents:** The diet may not provide enough calories or nutrients for healthy growth and development.

3. **People with a history of disordered eating:** This diet may trigger unhealthy behaviors or thought patterns related to food and body image.

4. **People with certain medical conditions:** Individuals with diabetes, kidney disease, liver disease, or other medical conditions should consult with their healthcare provider before starting this diet, as it may not be appropriate for their specific needs.

It's always a good idea to consult with a healthcare professional before starting any new diet or exercise program to ensure it is safe and appropriate for your individual needs and goals.

Recommendations For Those Considering The Diet

If you are considering the Metabolic Confusion Diet, here are some recommendations to help you get started:

1. **Consult with a healthcare professional:** Before starting any new diet or exercise plan, it's important to speak with a healthcare professional, especially if you have any pre-existing medical conditions or concerns.

2. **Plan and prepare meals in advance:** Meal planning and preparation can help you stick to the diet and avoid making unhealthy food choices when you are busy or on-the-go. Set aside time each week to plan and prepare your meals and snacks.

3. **Incorporate exercise:** Exercise is an important component of the diet and can help you achieve your weight loss and fitness goals. Consult with a fitness professional to determine the best types of exercise for your fitness level and goals.

4. **Keep track of your progress:** Keep track of your weight loss progress, as well as how you are feeling physically and emotionally. This can help you identify any areas of the diet that are working well for you, as well as areas that may

need improvement.

5. **Stay motivated:** Sticking to a diet can be challenging, but there are ways to stay motivated. Set realistic goals, reward yourself for achieving milestones, and enlist the support of family and friends.

Remember, the Metabolic Confusion Diet may not be suitable for everyone, so it's important to speak with a healthcare professional before starting the diet. Additionally, it's important to listen to your body and make adjustments as needed to ensure that you are meeting your nutritional needs and staying healthy.

CHAPTER TWO

Understanding Metabolism

Explanation Of Metabolism

Metabolism refers to the chemical processes that occur within the body to maintain life. It involves a complex series of reactions that break down food into usable energy and building blocks for the body's tissues and organs.

The metabolism is responsible for converting food into energy, which is used to power all bodily functions, including breathing, circulating blood, and repairing and growing tissues. It also helps to eliminate waste products and toxins from the body.

The metabolism can be divided into two main categories: catabolism and anabolism. Catabolism refers to the breakdown of complex molecules, such as carbohydrates, proteins, and fats, into smaller molecules that can be used by the body for energy. Anabolism, on the other hand, refers to the synthesis of complex molecules from smaller molecules, which is used to build and repair tissues and organs.

The rate of metabolism varies from person to person, and is influenced by a number of factors, including age, gender, genetics, body composition, and activity level. Generally speaking, the metabolism tends to slow down with age, which can contribute to weight gain and other health problems.

While the metabolism plays a crucial role in maintaining overall health and well-being, it is important to note that there is no single way to "boost" the metabolism or speed up weight loss. While certain foods, such as spicy foods and those high in protein, may temporarily increase metabolism, the most effective way to achieve sustainable weight loss is through a combination of healthy eating habits, regular exercise, and a balanced lifestyle.

Factors That Affect Metabolism

Metabolism is a complex process that involves the chemical reactions occurring in the body to maintain life. Many factors can affect a person's metabolism, including age, gender, body composition, genetics, hormones, diet, physical activity, and sleep.

As people age, their metabolism slows down, making it harder to maintain a healthy weight and increasing the risk of health problems. Men typically have a higher metabolic rate than women due to differences in body composition and hormonal factors. People with a higher muscle mass have a higher metabolism because muscle tissue is more metabolically active than fat tissue.

Genetics also play a role in determining a person's metabolic rate, and some individuals may be predisposed to a slower or faster metabolism. Hormones such as thyroid hormones and insulin have a significant impact on metabolism, and imbalances in these hormones can lead to a slower metabolic rate.

Diet can affect metabolism as well, as eating too few calories or skipping meals slows down metabolism, while eating a balanced diet with sufficient protein helps maintain a healthy metabolic rate. Regular physical activity, particularly resistance training, can increase muscle mass and boost metabolism. Lack of sleep or poor sleep quality can also disrupt hormones that regulate metabolism, leading to a slower metabolic rate.

Understanding the factors that affect metabolism is crucial to promoting overall health and maintaining a healthy weight. While some factors such as genetics are beyond our control, adopting healthy lifestyle habits such as regular exercise, a balanced diet, and adequate sleep can help support a healthy metabolism and improve overall well-being.

How The Metabolic Confusion Diet Impacts Metabolism

The Metabolic Confusion Diet is believed to impact metabolism by keeping it from becoming too accustomed to a specific type of diet. This is accomplished by constantly changing the types of foods and macronutrients consumed. By regularly changing the diet, the body is forced to continually adapt and adjust, which may help to increase the number of calories burned at rest, also known as basal metabolic rate (BMR).

The diet's cycling between different types of diets, such as high-protein, low-carbohydrate or low-fat, high-carbohydrate, is thought to stimulate the metabolism and prevent it from becoming stagnant. This constant variation in the types of diets and foods consumed is believed to help the body to continue burning calories and prevent it from plateauing.

The Metabolic Confusion Diet also emphasizes consuming whole, unprocessed foods, which can provide the body with the nutrients and energy it needs to function optimally. Additionally, the diet promotes regular exercise, which can help to increase muscle mass and improve overall metabolic rate. Muscle tissue is more metabolically active than fat tissue, meaning that it requires more energy (calories) to maintain.

While the Metabolic Confusion Diet may help boost metabolism and promote weight loss, it's important to note that it is a relatively new diet, and more research is needed to fully understand its effectiveness. It's essential to consult with a healthcare professional before starting any new diet or lifestyle change, especially if you have any underlying health conditions or concerns.

Four Phases Of The Metabolic Confusion Diet

The Metabolic Confusion Diet consists of four phases, each with its own specific guidelines and goals. These phases are designed to promote weight loss, boost metabolism, and improve overall health. Here is an overview of each phase:

1. **Phase One: Reset** - This phase lasts for two weeks and involves a low-carbohydrate, high-protein diet. The goal is to reset the body's metabolism by reducing insulin levels and

promoting fat burning.

2. **Phase Two: Rotate** - This phase lasts for six weeks and involves cycling between high-carbohydrate, low-fat days and low-carbohydrate, high-fat days. The goal is to keep the metabolism guessing and prevent it from becoming stagnant.

3. **Phase Three: Recharge** - This phase lasts for two weeks and involves a high-carbohydrate, low-protein diet. The goal is to replenish glycogen stores in the muscles and provide the body with energy for exercise.

4. **Phase Four: Lifestyle** - This phase is ongoing and involves following a healthy, balanced diet that emphasizes whole, unprocessed foods and regular exercise. The goal is to maintain weight loss and promote overall health and well-being.

Each phase of the Metabolic Confusion Diet is designed to build on the previous phase and gradually transition the body to a healthy, sustainable lifestyle. It's important to follow the guidelines of each phase carefully and consult with a healthcare professional before starting the diet, especially if you have any underlying health conditions or concerns.

Overview Of Each Phase

1. **Phase One: Reset** - During this two-week phase, the focus is on reducing insulin levels and promoting fat burning. This is achieved through a low-carbohydrate, high-protein diet,

which helps to control blood sugar levels and increase satiety. You'll consume lean protein sources, such as chicken, fish, and turkey, along with non-starchy vegetables, healthy fats, and limited amounts of low-glycemic fruits and carbohydrates. This phase is designed to reset your metabolism and prepare your body for the following phases.

2. **Phase Two: Rotate** - This six-week phase involves cycling between high-carbohydrate, low-fat days and low-carbohydrate, high-fat days. This approach helps to keep your metabolism guessing and prevent it from adapting to a specific type of diet. On high-carbohydrate days, you'll consume healthy carbohydrates, such as fruits, vegetables, and whole grains, along with lean protein and limited amounts of healthy fats. On low-carbohydrate days, you'll consume healthy fats, such as nuts, seeds, and avocado, along with lean protein and non-starchy vegetables. This phase is designed to further increase fat burning and promote weight loss.

3. **Phase Three: Recharge** - This two-week phase involves a high-carbohydrate, low-protein diet, which helps to replenish glycogen stores in the muscles and provide energy for exercise. During this phase, you'll consume healthy carbohydrates, such as fruits, vegetables, and whole grains, along with limited amounts of protein and healthy fats. This phase is designed to provide the body with the energy it needs

for physical activity and improve exercise performance.

4. **Phase Four: Lifestyle** - This ongoing phase involves following a healthy, balanced diet that emphasizes whole, unprocessed foods and regular exercise. The goal is to maintain weight loss and promote overall health and well-being. During this phase, you'll continue to consume lean protein, healthy fats, and a variety of fruits and vegetables while limiting processed foods, sugar, and refined carbohydrates. This phase is designed to help you establish healthy habits for life and prevent weight regain.

Overall, the Metabolic Confusion Diet is a four-phase approach to weight loss and improved health that is based on scientific principles of metabolism and nutrition. It's important to follow the guidelines of each phase carefully and consult with a healthcare professional before starting the diet, especially if you have any underlying health conditions or concerns.

Benefits Of Each Phase

1. **Phase One: Reset** - In this phase, the body is reset by reducing carbohydrate intake and focusing on consuming whole, nutrient-dense foods. This may help to improve insulin sensitivity, which is important for maintaining stable blood sugar levels and preventing weight gain. Additionally, reducing inflammation in the body can improve overall health and reduce the risk of chronic diseases. The focus on whole

regain, and reduce the risk of chronic diseases. By focusing on whole, nutrient-dense foods and maintaining a healthy balance of macronutrients, this phase can also improve overall nutrition and provide important micronutrients.

It's important to note that the benefits of the Metabolic Confusion Diet may vary from person to person and there is limited scientific research on its effectiveness and safety. It's important to follow the guidelines of each phase carefully, listen to your body, and consult with a healthcare professional before starting any new diet or exercise program.

Foods To Eat And Avoid During Each Phase

1. Phase One: Reset

Foods to eat:

- Lean proteins (e.g. chicken, fish, turkey, tofu)
- Non-starchy vegetables (e.g. broccoli, spinach, cauliflower, zucchini)
- Low glycemic index fruits (e.g. berries, apples, pears)
- Healthy fats (e.g. avocado, nuts, seeds, olive oil)

Foods to avoid:

- Processed foods (e.g. packaged snacks, fast food)
- Refined carbohydrates (e.g. white bread, pasta, rice)

- Sugary drinks (e.g. soda, juice, sweetened coffee or tea)
- High glycemic index fruits (e.g. bananas, pineapple, mango)

2. Phase Two: Rotate

Foods to eat:

- Complex carbohydrates (e.g. sweet potatoes, quinoa, brown rice)
- Lean proteins (e.g. grass-fed beef, eggs, lentils)
- Healthy fats (e.g. coconut oil, nut butter, chia seeds)
- Non-starchy vegetables (e.g. kale, asparagus, brussels sprouts)

Foods to avoid:

- Simple carbohydrates (e.g. candy, pastries, white bread)
- Processed foods (e.g. frozen meals, packaged snacks)
- High glycemic index carbohydrates (e.g. white potatoes, white rice, corn)
- Fatty meats (e.g. bacon, sausage, fried chicken)

3. Phase Three: Recharge

Foods to eat:

- Healthy carbohydrates (e.g. sweet potatoes, bananas, quinoa)
- Lean proteins (e.g. grilled chicken, wild-caught

salmon, beans)

- Healthy fats (e.g. avocado, nuts, seeds)
- Non-starchy vegetables (e.g. leafy greens, peppers, cucumbers)

Foods to avoid:

- Processed carbohydrates (e.g. white bread, sugary cereals, candy)
- Fried foods (e.g. french fries, onion rings, fried chicken)
- Sugary drinks (e.g. soda, sweetened coffee drinks)
- High-fat dairy products (e.g. full-fat cheese, ice cream)

4. Phase Four: Lifestyle

Foods to eat:

- Whole, nutrient-dense foods (e.g. fruits, vegetables, whole grains, lean proteins)
- Healthy fats (e.g. avocado, nuts, seeds, olive oil)
- Low-fat dairy products (e.g. skim milk, low-fat yogurt)
- Limited amounts of processed foods and added sugars

Foods to avoid:

- Highly processed foods (e.g. packaged snacks, fast food)
- Sugary drinks (e.g. soda, sweetened coffee drinks)

- High-fat meats (e.g. bacon, sausage, fatty cuts of beef)

- Excess amounts of saturated and trans fats (e.g. fried foods, processed meats)

Remember that the foods to eat and avoid may vary based on individual preferences and dietary restrictions. It's important to consult with a healthcare professional and/or registered dietitian before starting any new diet or making significant changes to your current eating habits.

CHAPTER THREE

Calorie Cycling

Explanation Of Calorie Cycling

Calorie cycling is a dietary technique where you alternate between days of high-calorie intake and days of low-calorie intake. The purpose of calorie cycling is to promote weight loss by preventing your metabolism from getting used to a set calorie intake, which can lead to a plateau in weight loss.

The concept behind calorie cycling is to keep your body guessing and prevent it from adapting to a consistent calorie intake, which can cause your metabolism to slow down over time. For example, if you consistently consume a low-calorie diet for an extended period, your body will eventually adapt by lowering your metabolism, making it harder to lose weight.

With calorie cycling, you may consume more calories than your body needs on high-calorie days, and then consume fewer calories on low-calorie days. This can help keep your metabolism elevated, allowing your body to continue burning calories and promoting weight loss.

However, it's important to note that calorie cycling should be done with caution and under the guidance of a healthcare professional or registered dietitian. It's essential to make sure you're still consuming enough calories to support your body's needs, even on low-calorie days, and that you're getting all the nutrients your body needs to function properly. Additionally, calorie cycling may not be appropriate for everyone, especially those with a history of disordered eating or certain medical conditions.

How Calorie Cycling Impacts Weight Loss

Calorie cycling is a dietary technique that involves alternating between days of high and low calorie intake. This approach can help prevent weight loss plateaus and improve fat loss by keeping the metabolism elevated and preventing it from adapting to a consistent calorie intake.

On days of low-calorie intake, the body enters a calorie deficit, which causes it to burn stored fat for energy, leading to weight loss. On high-calorie days, the body consumes more calories than it needs, which helps prevent the metabolism from slowing down and promotes muscle growth.

Calorie cycling can be an effective weight loss strategy because it helps to keep the body guessing and prevents it from becoming too accustomed to a specific calorie intake. This approach can also help prevent hunger and cravings associated with sustained calorie restriction.

However, it is essential to approach calorie cycling with caution and seek the advice of a healthcare professional or registered dietitian to ensure that you are still consuming enough calories to meet your body's needs and getting all the necessary nutrients for proper functioning.

Additionally, calorie cycling may not be appropriate for everyone, particularly those with certain medical conditions or a history of disordered eating.

How To Calculate Calorie Needs And Set Up A Calorie Cycling Plan

To calculate your calorie needs for a calorie cycling plan, you will first need to determine your daily calorie requirements. This can be done using an online calculator or by consulting with a healthcare professional or registered dietitian.

Once you have determined your daily calorie requirements, you can begin to set up your calorie cycling plan. A typical calorie cycling plan may involve alternating between high-calorie days and low-calorie days. The low-calorie days should still provide enough energy to support normal bodily functions and physical activity, while the high-calorie days should provide enough energy to promote muscle growth and prevent the metabolism from slowing down.

A sample calorie cycling plan might involve consuming 1,500 calories on low-calorie days and 2,500 calories on high-calorie days. This would result in an average daily calorie intake of 2,000 calories, which may be appropriate for weight loss depending on your individual needs and goals.

It is important to note that calorie cycling plans should be tailored to individual needs and goals and should take into account factors such as age, gender, height, weight, activity level, and overall health status.

In addition to calorie cycling, it is also important to focus on consuming a balanced and nutritious diet that includes a variety of whole foods such as fruits, vegetables, lean proteins, whole grains, and healthy fats. Staying hydrated and engaging in regular physical activity can also support weight loss and overall health.

CHAPTER FOUR

*Nutritional Guidelines for the
Metabolic Confusion Diet*

Overview Of Macronutrients And Micronutrients

Macronutrients are nutrients that are needed by the body in large amounts to provide energy and support bodily functions. They include carbohydrates, proteins, and fats.

Carbohydrates are the body's primary source of energy, and they are found in foods such as bread, pasta, rice, fruits, and vegetables. Proteins are important for building and repairing tissues, as well as supporting immune function and producing enzymes and hormones. Foods that are high in protein include meat, fish, eggs, dairy products, and legumes. Fats are necessary for the absorption of certain vitamins, as well as for hormone production and maintaining healthy skin and hair. Foods that are high in healthy fats include nuts, seeds, oils, fatty fish, and avocados.

Micronutrients, on the other hand, are needed by the body in smaller amounts, but they are still essential for good health. They include vitamins and minerals, which are important for maintaining strong bones, supporting immune function, and helping the body convert food into energy.

Vitamins are organic compounds that the body needs in small amounts to function properly. They are found in a variety of foods, such as fruits, vegetables, whole grains, dairy products, and meats. For example, vitamin C is found in citrus fruits, vitamin A in carrots, and vitamin D in fatty fish.

Minerals are inorganic compounds that are needed in small amounts to maintain good health. They are found in a variety of foods, such as leafy greens, whole grains, nuts, and meats. Examples of important minerals include calcium, which is important for building strong bones and teeth, and iron, which is needed for healthy red blood cells.

Recommended Daily Intake Of Each Nutrient

Carbohydrates: The recommended daily intake of carbohydrates varies depending on age, gender, activity level, and other factors. In general, it is recommended that adults get 45-65% of their daily calories from carbohydrates, with a minimum of 130 grams per day.

Proteins: The recommended daily intake of protein also varies depending on age, gender, activity level, and other factors. In general, it is recommended that adults get 10-35% of their daily calories from protein, with a minimum of 0.8 grams of protein per kilogram of body weight per day.

Fats: The recommended daily intake of fat also varies

depending on age, gender, activity level, and other factors. In general, it is recommended that adults get 20-35% of their daily calories from fat, with a focus on consuming healthy fats such as monounsaturated and polyunsaturated fats.

Vitamins: The recommended daily intake of vitamins also varies depending on age, gender, and other factors. The recommended daily intake levels for each vitamin can be found on the Nutrition Facts label on food packaging or through reputable health sources.

Minerals: The recommended daily intake of minerals also varies depending on age, gender, and other factors. The recommended daily intake levels for each mineral can be found on the Nutrition Facts label on food packaging or through reputable health sources.

It's important to note that individual nutrient needs can vary based on factors such as age, gender, weight, and health status. Consult with a healthcare provider or registered dietitian to determine your specific nutrient needs.

Tips For Meeting Nutritional Needs While Following The Diet

Here are some tips for making sure you're meeting your nutritional needs while following the diet:

1. **Plan ahead:** Planning your meals in advance can help ensure that you're getting a variety of nutrient-dense foods. This can also help you stay on track with your calorie and nutrient goals for each phase of the diet.

2. **Focus on nutrient-dense foods:** Nutrient-dense foods are those that are high in nutrients but relatively low in calories. These include fruits, vegetables, whole grains, lean proteins, and healthy fats. Including a variety of these foods in your meals can help ensure you're getting all the necessary vitamins and minerals.

3. **Monitor portion sizes:** Even healthy foods can contribute to weight gain if consumed in excess. Be mindful of portion sizes and aim to eat until you're satisfied, not overly full.

4. **Use supplements if necessary:** While it's best to get nutrients from whole foods whenever possible, supplements can be helpful if you're struggling to meet your nutrient needs. Consult with a healthcare professional before starting any new supplements.

5. **Stay hydrated:** Drinking enough water is important for overall health and can also help with weight loss. Aim to drink at least 8 cups of water per day, and consider drinking more if you're physically active.

6. **Be mindful of alcohol and sugary drinks:** These beverages can be high in calories and offer little nutritional value. Limit your intake and opt for healthier alternatives such as water, herbal tea, or low-calorie beverages.

7. **Consult with a registered dietitian:** If you're struggling to meet your nutrient needs while

following the Metabolic Confusion Diet, a registered dietitian can help you create a personalized meal plan that meets your specific needs. They can also provide guidance on supplement use and help ensure you're getting all the necessary nutrients for optimal health.

Meal Planning Tips

Meal planning is a crucial aspect of the Metabolic Confusion Diet. Proper planning ensures that individuals consume the right foods in the right amounts, which helps them achieve their weight loss goals while meeting their nutritional needs. Here are some tips for meal planning on the Metabolic Confusion Diet:

1. **Start with a plan:** Before you start your diet, make a meal plan for each phase of the diet. Include a variety of healthy foods that meet your nutritional needs and calorie requirements for each phase.

2. **Focus on whole, nutrient-dense foods:** Incorporate plenty of fruits, vegetables, whole grains, lean proteins, and healthy fats into your meals. These foods provide essential nutrients and help you feel full and satisfied.

3. **Be mindful of portion sizes:** While the diet doesn't require calorie counting, it's important to pay attention to portion sizes to avoid overeating. Use measuring cups and spoons or a food scale to ensure you're eating the right amount of food.

4. **Prep meals in advance:** Preparing meals in advance saves time and ensures that you always have healthy options on hand. Try meal prepping on weekends for the week ahead.

5. **Experiment with recipes:** Don't be afraid to try new recipes and experiment with different flavors and textures. This helps you avoid boredom and makes mealtime more enjoyable.

By following these tips, individuals can plan and prepare nutritious meals that support their weight loss goals while following the Metabolic Confusion Diet.

15 Diet Sample Meal Plan

Day 1:

Breakfast: Greek yogurt with mixed berries and walnuts

Lunch: Turkey and hummus wrap with avocado and cucumber

Dinner: Baked salmon with quinoa and roasted asparagus

Day 2:

Breakfast: Spinach and feta omelet with whole grain toast

Lunch: Chicken and veggie stir-fry with brown rice

Dinner: Grilled chicken with sweet potato and green beans

Day 3:

Breakfast: Protein smoothie with banana, spinach, and almond butter

Lunch: Tuna salad with mixed greens and tomato

Dinner: Beef and broccoli stir-fry with brown rice

Day 4:

Breakfast: Overnight oats with blueberries and almond milk

Lunch: Grilled chicken salad with mixed greens and avocado

Dinner: Pork chops with roasted Brussels sprouts and sweet potato

Day 5:

Breakfast: Scrambled eggs with spinach and tomato

Lunch: Quinoa and black bean salad with avocado and tomato

Dinner: Baked chicken with roasted carrots and brown rice

Day 6:

Breakfast: Greek yogurt with sliced banana and granola

Lunch: Turkey and veggie wrap with hummus

Dinner: Grilled salmon with quinoa and roasted zucchini

Day 7:

Breakfast: Protein smoothie with mango, spinach, and Greek yogurt

Lunch: Chicken Caesar salad with mixed greens and tomato

Dinner: Beef and veggie stir-fry with brown rice

Day 8:

Breakfast: Scrambled eggs with mushroom and tomato

Lunch: Tuna and avocado salad with mixed greens

Dinner: Baked chicken with roasted broccoli and sweet potato

Day 9:

Breakfast: Overnight oats with raspberries and almond milk

Lunch: Grilled chicken and veggie kebab with brown rice

Dinner: Pork chops with roasted green beans and quinoa

Day 10:

Breakfast: Protein smoothie with peach, spinach, and almond butter

Lunch: Turkey and hummus wrap with cucumber and tomato

Dinner: Baked salmon with roasted Brussels sprouts and quinoa

Day 11:

Breakfast: Greek yogurt with mixed berries and granola

Lunch: Chicken and veggie stir-fry with brown rice

Dinner: Grilled chicken with roasted sweet potato and asparagus

Day 12:

Breakfast: Spinach and feta omelet with whole grain toast

Lunch: Tuna salad with mixed greens and avocado

Dinner: Beef and broccoli stir-fry with brown rice

Day 13:

Breakfast: Protein smoothie with banana, spinach, and almond butter

Lunch: Grilled chicken salad with mixed greens and avocado

Dinner: Pork chops with roasted Brussels sprouts and sweet potato

Day 14:

Breakfast: Overnight oats with blueberries and almond milk

Lunch: Quinoa and black bean salad with avocado and tomato

Dinner: Baked chicken with roasted carrots and brown rice

Day 15:

Breakfast: Scrambled eggs with spinach and tomato

Lunch: Turkey and veggie wrap with hummus

Dinner: Grilled salmon with quinoa and roasted zucchini

CHAPTER FIVE

*Exercise and the Metabolic
Confusion Diet*

Exercise is an important component of the Metabolic Confusion Diet, as it helps to increase metabolism and improve overall health and fitness. Here are some ways that exercise can be incorporated into the diet:

1. **Resistance training:** Resistance training, such as weight lifting, can help to build lean muscle mass, which in turn increases metabolism. Aim to include resistance training exercises at least two to three times per week.

2. **Cardiovascular exercise:** Cardiovascular exercise, such as running or cycling, can help to burn calories and improve cardiovascular health. Try to include cardiovascular exercise for at least 30 minutes, three to four times per week.

3. **HIIT workouts:** High-intensity interval training (HIIT) workouts involve short bursts of intense exercise followed by periods of rest. These types of workouts have been shown to increase metabolism and burn fat. Consider incorporating HIIT workouts into

your exercise routine once or twice a week.

4. **Active lifestyle:** In addition to structured exercise, try to maintain an active lifestyle by walking more, taking the stairs instead of the elevator, and engaging in other forms of physical activity throughout the day.

It's important to note that while exercise can be beneficial for weight loss and overall health, it's not necessary to follow a strict exercise routine to see results on the Metabolic Confusion Diet. The focus should be on finding physical activities that are enjoyable and sustainable for the long term.

Benefits Of Exercise While Following The Diet

Incorporating exercise into your routine while following the Metabolic Confusion Diet can provide numerous benefits. Exercise can help to increase your metabolism and promote fat loss. It also helps to build and tone muscle, which can give your body a more defined and sculpted appearance.

In addition to the physical benefits, exercise can also improve your mood and reduce stress levels. Regular physical activity has been shown to release endorphins, which are feel-good hormones that can help to reduce feelings of anxiety and depression.

Another benefit of exercise while following the Metabolic Confusion Diet is that it can help to prevent weight loss plateaus. Plateaus can occur when your body adjusts to your calorie intake and activity level, which can slow down weight loss progress. Incorporating regular exercise into your routine can help to keep your body challenged and prevent plateaus from occurring.

It's important to note that while exercise can be beneficial for weight loss and overall health, it's not necessary to follow a rigorous exercise routine while following the Metabolic Confusion Diet. Simply adding moderate physical activity, such as brisk walking, yoga, or strength training, can provide significant benefits. It's important to listen to your body and not overexert yourself, especially if you're new to exercise or have any health concerns.

How To Incorporate Exercise Into The Diet Plan

Incorporating exercise into the Metabolic Confusion Diet plan can enhance the weight loss process and improve overall health. The American College of Sports Medicine recommends at least 150 minutes of moderate-intensity exercise or 75 minutes of vigorous-intensity exercise per week for adults.

The following are some tips on how to incorporate exercise into the diet plan:

1. **Start slow and gradually increase intensity:** It is essential to begin with low to moderate-intensity exercises, such as brisk walking, jogging, or cycling, and gradually increase intensity as the body adapts.

2. **Mix up cardio and strength training:**

Incorporating a combination of cardio and strength training exercises can help build lean muscle and burn fat. Cardio exercises include running, cycling, swimming, and dancing, while strength training can involve using weights, resistance bands, or bodyweight exercises like squats and push-ups.

3. **Schedule exercise sessions:** Planning and scheduling exercise sessions into the daily routine can help ensure consistency and adherence to the workout plan.

4. **Find an exercise partner:** Having a workout partner can provide motivation, accountability, and support during the weight loss journey.

5. **Be flexible:** Life can be unpredictable, and there may be days when it's difficult to fit in a full workout. On those days, aim to incorporate some physical activity into the routine, like taking a short walk or doing a few sets of push-ups.

By incorporating exercise into the Metabolic Confusion Diet plan, individuals can accelerate weight loss, improve overall health, and maintain long-term weight management.

CHAPTER SIX

Recipes for Metabolic
Confusion Diet

Chicken and Broccoli Stir-Fry

Ingredients:

- 1 pound boneless, skinless chicken breast, sliced into thin strips
- 2 tablespoons coconut oil
- 1 tablespoon minced garlic
- 1 tablespoon minced ginger
- 2 cups broccoli florets
- 1 red bell pepper, sliced into thin strips
- 1 tablespoon soy sauce
- 1 tablespoon hoisin sauce

Instructions:

1. Heat a large skillet over medium-high heat and add the coconut oil.

2. Add the chicken, garlic, and ginger to the skillet and cook until the chicken is browned and cooked through, about 5-7 minutes.

3. Add the broccoli and bell pepper to the skillet and cook for an additional 3-5 minutes, until the vegetables are tender-crisp.

4. Stir in the soy sauce and hoisin sauce, then serve.

Greek Yogurt Parfait

Ingredients:

- 1 cup plain Greek yogurt
- 1/2 cup mixed berries
- 1/4 cup chopped nuts
- 1 tablespoon honey

Instructions:

1. In a small bowl or jar, layer the Greek yogurt, mixed berries, and chopped nuts.

2. Drizzle with honey and serve.

Turkey and Sweet Potato Chili

Ingredients:

- 1 pound ground turkey
- 2 tablespoons olive oil
- 1 onion, diced
- 2 cloves garlic, minced
- 1 tablespoon chili powder
- 1 teaspoon cumin
- 1/2 teaspoon smoked paprika

- 1/4 teaspoon cayenne pepper
- 1 can diced tomatoes
- 1 can black beans, drained and rinsed
- 2 cups diced sweet potatoes
- 1 cup chicken broth

Instructions:

1. Heat the olive oil in a large pot over medium heat.

2. Add the onion and garlic and cook until softened, about 5 minutes.

3. Add the ground turkey and cook until browned, breaking it up with a spoon.

4. Stir in the chili powder, cumin, smoked paprika, and cayenne pepper.

5. Add the diced tomatoes (with their juice), black beans, sweet potatoes, and chicken broth to the pot.

6. Bring to a boil, then reduce heat and simmer until the sweet potatoes are tender, about 20-25 minutes.

Spinach and Feta Stuffed Chicken Breast

Ingredients:

- 4 boneless, skinless chicken breasts
- 1 cup frozen spinach, thawed and drained
- 1/2 cup crumbled feta cheese

- 2 cloves garlic, minced
- Salt and pepper

Instructions:

1. Preheat oven to 375°F.

2. Butterfly the chicken breasts by slicing horizontally through the center of each one, but not all the way through.

3. In a small bowl, mix together the spinach, feta cheese, garlic, salt, and pepper.

4. Spoon the spinach mixture onto one half of each chicken breast, then fold the other half over to enclose the filling.

5. Place the stuffed chicken breasts in a baking dish and bake for 25-30 minutes, until the chicken is cooked through.

Quinoa Salad with Grilled Chicken Ingredients:

Ingredients:

- 1 cup quinoa
- 2 cups water
- 1/4 cup olive oil
- 3 tbsp red wine vinegar
- 1 tbsp honey
- 1/4 tsp salt
- 1/4 tsp black pepper
- 2 cups chopped grilled chicken

- 1/2 cup chopped fresh parsley
- 1/2 cup chopped fresh mint
- 1/2 cup chopped fresh cilantro
- 1/2 cup chopped red onion
- 1 red bell pepper, chopped
- 1/2 cup crumbled feta cheese

Instructions:

1. Rinse the quinoa under cold water and drain well.

2. In a medium pot, bring the water to a boil. Add the quinoa and reduce heat to low. Cover and simmer for about 15-20 minutes, or until the water is absorbed and the quinoa is tender.

3. Fluff the quinoa with a fork and transfer it to a large bowl.

4. In a small bowl, whisk together the olive oil, red wine vinegar, honey, salt, and pepper.

5. Pour the dressing over the quinoa and toss to combine.

6. Add the grilled chicken, parsley, mint, cilantro, red onion, and bell pepper to the bowl.

7. Toss the salad well to combine all the ingredients.

8. Sprinkle the feta cheese over the top of the salad.

9. Serve the quinoa salad immediately, or store it in the fridge for up to 3 days.

Greek Yogurt Breakfast Bowl

Ingredients:

- 1 cup Greek yogurt
- 1/2 cup mixed berries
- 1/4 cup granola
- 1 tsp honey

Instructions:

1. In a bowl, add the Greek yogurt.
2. Top with mixed berries and granola.
3. Drizzle honey over the top.
4. Serve and enjoy.

Turkey and Sweet Potato Skillet

Ingredients:

- 1 lb ground turkey
- 1 large sweet potato, diced
- 1/2 onion, diced
- 1 bell pepper, diced
- 2 cloves garlic, minced
- 1 tsp chili powder
- 1 tsp cumin

- 1/2 tsp paprika
- Salt and pepper to taste
- 1 tbsp olive oil

Instructions:

1. Heat the olive oil in a skillet over medium heat.

2. Add the onion, bell pepper, and garlic. Cook until the onion is translucent.

3. Add the ground turkey and cook until browned.

4. Add the sweet potato, chili powder, cumin, paprika, salt, and pepper. Stir well.

5. Cover the skillet and let it cook until the sweet potatoes are tender.

6. Serve and enjoy.

Grilled Chicken with Roasted Vegetables

Ingredients:

- 4 boneless, skinless chicken breasts
- 2 bell peppers, sliced
- 2 zucchinis, sliced
- 1 red onion, sliced
- 1 tsp garlic powder
- 1 tsp onion powder
- 1 tsp paprika
- Salt and pepper to taste

- 2 tbsp olive oil

Instructions:

1. Preheat the grill to medium-high heat.

2. In a large bowl, add the sliced bell peppers, zucchinis, and red onion.

3. Drizzle the vegetables with olive oil and sprinkle with garlic powder, onion powder, paprika, salt, and pepper.

4. Toss to coat the vegetables evenly.

5. Grill the chicken until cooked through.

6. Roast the vegetables in the oven at 400°F for 20-25 minutes or until they are tender and slightly browned.

7. Serve the chicken with the roasted vegetables and enjoy.

Shrimp and Broccoli Stir-Fry

Ingredients:

- 1 lb shrimp, peeled and deveined

- 4 cups broccoli florets

- 1 red bell pepper, sliced

- 2 cloves garlic, minced

- 2 tbsp soy sauce

- 1 tbsp honey

- 1 tbsp olive oil

Instructions:

1. Heat the olive oil in a large skillet over medium heat.

2. Add the garlic and cook until fragrant.

3. Add the shrimp and cook until pink.

4. Remove the shrimp from the skillet and set aside.

5. In the same skillet, add the broccoli and red bell pepper. Cook until tender.

6. In a small bowl, mix together the soy sauce and honey.

7. Add the shrimp back to the skillet and pour the soy sauce mixture over everything.

8. Stir until everything is coated and heated through.

9. Serve and enjoy.

Tuna Salad Lettuce Wraps

Ingredients:

- 2 cans tuna, drained
- 1/2 cup plain Greek yogurt
- 1/4 cup chopped celery
- 1/4 cup chopped red onion
- 2 tbsp chopped fresh parsley

- Salt and pepper to taste

- 4 large lettuce leaves

Instructions:

1. In a large bowl, mix together the tuna, Greek yogurt, celery, red onion, parsley, salt, Scoop the tuna salad mixture onto each lettuce leaf.

2. Sprinkle some additional chopped green onions and sesame seeds over the top for garnish.

3. Serve immediately and enjoy your delicious and nutritious Tuna Salad Lettuce Wraps!

4. Optional: You can also add sliced avocado or cucumber to the lettuce wraps for additional flavor and nutrition.

Note: This recipe makes about 4 servings, but can easily be scaled up or down to fit your needs.

Baked salmon with roasted vegetables

Ingredients:

- 4 oz salmon fillet

- 1 cup mixed vegetables (such as broccoli, carrots, and bell peppers)

- 1 tbsp olive oil

- Salt and pepper to taste

Instructions:

1. Preheat the oven to 375°F.

2. Place the salmon fillet on a baking sheet and season with salt and pepper.

3. Toss the mixed vegetables with olive oil, salt, and pepper, and spread them around the salmon on the baking sheet.

4. Bake for 15-20 minutes or until the salmon is cooked through and the vegetables are tender.

Chicken and vegetable stir-fry

Ingredients:

- 4 oz chicken breast, sliced

- 1 cup mixed vegetables (such as broccoli, bell peppers, and mushrooms)

- 1 tbsp olive oil

- 2 cloves garlic, minced

- 1 tsp grated ginger

- Salt and pepper to taste

Instructions:

1. Heat the olive oil in a large skillet over medium-high heat.

2. Add the chicken and stir-fry for 2-3 minutes until lightly browned.

3. Add the mixed vegetables, garlic, and ginger, and continue to stir-fry for 3-4 minutes until the vegetables are tender and the chicken is

cooked through.

4. Season with salt and pepper to taste.

Lentil soup with spinach and carrots

Ingredients:

- 1 cup lentils, rinsed and drained
- 4 cups vegetable broth
- 1 cup chopped spinach
- 1 cup chopped carrots
- 1 tbsp olive oil
- 1 onion, chopped
- 2 cloves garlic, minced
- 1 tsp cumin
- Salt and pepper to taste

Instructions:

1. Heat the olive oil in a large pot over medium-high heat.

2. Add the onion and garlic and sauté for 2-3 minutes until softened.

3. Add the lentils, vegetable broth, cumin, salt, and pepper, and bring to a boil.

4. Reduce the heat to low and simmer for 20-25 minutes until the lentils are tender.

5. Add the chopped spinach and carrots and

cook for an additional 5-10 minutes until the vegetables are tender.

Turkey and sweet potato chili

Ingredients:

- 4 oz ground turkey
- 1 cup diced sweet potato
- 1 cup diced tomatoes
- 1 cup black beans, rinsed and drained
- 1 onion, chopped
- 1 clove garlic, minced
- 1 tbsp olive oil
- 1 tsp chili powder
- Salt and pepper to taste

Instructions:

1. Heat the olive oil in a large pot over medium-high heat.

2. Add the onion and garlic and sauté for 2-3 minutes until softened.

3. Add the ground turkey and cook until browned.

4. Add the sweet potato, diced tomatoes, black beans, chili powder, salt, and pepper, and stir to combine.

5. Bring the mixture to a boil, then reduce the heat and simmer for 20-25 minutes until the sweet potato is tender.

Mediterranean-style chicken and vegetable skewers:

Ingredients:

- 1 pound boneless, skinless chicken breasts, cut into 1-inch cubes

- 1 red bell pepper, cut into 1-inch pieces

- 1 yellow bell pepper, cut into 1-inch pieces

- 1 red onion, cut into 1-inch pieces

- 1 zucchini, sliced into 1/2-inch rounds

- 2 tablespoons olive oil

- 2 tablespoons balsamic vinegar

- 1 tablespoon lemon juice

- 1 tablespoon chopped fresh rosemary

- 1 tablespoon chopped fresh thyme

- Salt and pepper to taste

- Skewers

Instructions:

1. Preheat grill to medium-high heat.

2. In a bowl, whisk together the olive oil, balsamic vinegar, lemon juice, rosemary, thyme, salt, and pepper.

3. Thread the chicken, bell peppers, onion, and zucchini onto the skewers.

4. Brush the skewers with the marinade.

5. Grill the skewers for 10-12 minutes, turning occasionally, until the chicken is cooked through and the vegetables are slightly charred.

6. Serve hot and enjoy!

CONCLUSION

The Metabolic Confusion Diet is a flexible and effective way to promote weight loss and overall health. By cycling between different calorie and nutrient ratios, the body is challenged and forced to adapt, which can lead to increased metabolic rate and fat burning. However, it is important to approach this diet with caution and ensure that nutritional needs are being met. It is also important to incorporate exercise into the plan to maximize results and improve overall health.

While the Metabolic Confusion Diet may not be suitable for everyone, it can be a valuable tool for those looking to lose weight and improve their health. By following the tips and guidelines outlined in this guide, individuals can successfully implement this diet into their lifestyle and achieve their weight loss goals. As with any diet or lifestyle change, it is important to consult with a healthcare professional before starting and to listen to your body throughout the process.